TAKE CHARGE

Take Charge
Weight Control for Tweens

iUniverse books may be ordered through booksellers or by contacting:

iUniverse
1663 Liberty Drive
Bloomington, IN 47403
www.iuniverse.com
1-800-Authors (1-800-288-4677)

Because of the dynamic nature of the Internet, any Web addresses or links contained in this book may have changed since publication and may no longer be valid. The views expressed in this work are solely those of the author and do not necessarily reflect the views of the publisher, and the publisher hereby disclaims any responsibility for them.

ISBN: 978-1-4401-2190-6 (pbk)
ISBN: 978-1-4401-2191-3 (ebk)

Printed in the United States of America

iUniverse rev. date: 2/6/2009

Contents

I am indebted to Dr. Jane McGoldrick and Dr. William Cottrell for some specific information. Thane Puissegur has given me support and made helpful comments on the manuscript, and Sharon Stewart provided invaluable editorial help. Of course, any errors are mine alone.

Important Note

This book is not a medical text. It is intended as a general guide to nutrition and exercise that tweens can use productively. The author and publisher take no responsibility for any misuse of this information. Specific questions about weight control should be directed to a physician, dietitian, or other professional.

A Note for Teachers and Parents

You may have provided this workbook because you are concerned about a child's weight. Please make the workbook available without much comment, and do not use it for giving children assignments. I have emphasized to readers that while many factors influence eating, individuals are responsible for their own "bottom line" in weight control. In coming to terms with their weight issues, young people should use the book as a sort of personal diary, even as a secret one. If your child wants to share it with you or to ask advice, fine! You can be very helpful in many ways—in fact, children are more successful in controlling their weight when the whole family is involved in planning meals and exercising—but any sharing of this book should be voluntary. If you would like to expand your own knowledge about weight control, please refer to the For Further Reading section at the end of the book.

The Problem of Weight

Do you ever worry about your weight? If so, you're not alone. Today it seems as if everybody talks about the "obesity epidemic" and worries about its effect on young people. Parents and teachers want to help. As a result, maybe things have changed a little in your school or city. In some schools, junk food has been replaced by salad bars, and it's harder to find sugary soft drinks. You may be getting more exercise at school, too.

Those changes can help a lot, but you may have trouble controlling your weight anyway. You may eat too much, or too much of the wrong foods, outside of school. You may eat too much fast food. You may ride in a car or school bus when you could be walking. All those things can lead to gaining weight.

In modern times, it's all too easy to gain weight, and it's hard to lose it. You've probably heard many ideas for avoiding obesity—"Ban soft drinks in schools!" "Increase time for physical education!" "Cut down on TV time!" "Eat fewer carbs!" "Eat less protein!" "Drink more water!" "Wash your neck!" (I'm kidding.)

Most of the suggestions are aimed at influences in your surroundings. Very often fast-food restaurants are blamed, because many fast foods are high in calories or have too much fat. Soft-drink manufacturers are blamed for selling sugary drinks. Advertisers are blamed for making fattening foods and drinks hard to resist. Parents and schools are blamed for not providing the right kind of meals. The government is blamed for not setting and enforcing standards. And so on.

It's very easy to think, "It's their fault, not mine. I'm gaining weight because I can't help it." Think about that, and be honest with yourself. Yes, it can be hard to keep your weight where it ought to be, but no one is forcing you to eat too much. You can make choices every day that will help you stay at a good weight for your height. You will look better and feel better.

Your doctor or school nurse can help you by telling you how much you weigh and giving you advice about good foods and exercise. Making the right choices is your job, though. It's important for you to take charge of your weight yourself.

You may have seen books, magazine articles, or online sites about weight control. Usually, they simply give you a lot of information and tell you what to do. This book is different. Each chapter begins with an activity that will help you learn something about weight control or about yourself. Then you can decide how to apply what you've learned. For instance, for one activity you compare cereals in a supermarket. Afterward, you can decide how to use the comparison. It's all up to you!

Don't even try to rush through the book. Instead, do the activities and fill in the tables and answers gradually. Take it one step at a time, but do keep taking the steps. Each day, do at least one thing—continue an activity that lasts for a week or more, or try a new activity that can be carried out in a few minutes. If you really don't want to do an activity, skip to the next one. But I hope you will try most of them, to find out what works best for you. You may want to spend weeks or months working your way through the book.

Not every strategy works for everyone. If you try an activity for a week or so and it doesn't help you, go on to another. By the time you finish this book, you will have learned many things about weight control, and about yourself. That will help you use the methods that work for you.

Many of the activities contain tables and blanks to be filled in. Some show sample answers in *italics*. Use the samples as a guide for adding your own answers.

This book is your own personal record of how you are taking charge of your weight. You may want to hide it under your mattress, and not show it to anyone! Or you may decide to show it to someone who can help you. Making that choice is part of taking charge.

What's Holding You Back?

Do you ever think, "I could lose weight, if only . . ." If only what? Is something or someone causing you to eat too much, or to exercise too little? If there is, maybe you can change that situation.

Chances are, though, that you have to make some changes in yourself instead. You can learn more about food so you find it easier to eat less fattening things. You can start enjoying exercises that will help you.

Sometimes we gain weight without knowing why it happened. If you feel unhappy or anxious, you may tend to eat too much. That can make you feel better for a little while. Or you may stay indoors rather than going out and getting exercise. Eating too much and moving too little can lead to weight gain.

If you often feel sad, lonely, or upset, get some help. Talk to someone you trust. A teacher, counselor, parent or grandparent, or other trusted adult may be able to help you deal with feelings that may affect your weight.

Test yourself

Before going farther, answer the following questions. Some have right answers, and others do not.

1.   What is your favorite snack? _____

2.   If a 2″ cookie has 100 calories, how many calories are in a 4″ cookie of the same kind and thickness? _____

3.   How far can you walk in 20 minutes if you walk 3 miles per hour? _____

4.   How much sleep do people your age need every night? _____

5.   What is the least fattening cereal you know about? _____

6.   Why is tofu a healthy food? _____

7.   How much milk should you drink every day? _____

8.   Does swimming or walking use up more calories a minute? _____

9.   Do you eat breakfast every day? _____

When you have finished the book, you will have another chance to answer the questions.

How much should you weigh?

It is hard to know exactly what you should weigh. Start by looking at your face and body in a full-length mirror. Do you look fat or thin? As a general guide to what you should weigh, measure your height and use the following table.

Height (inches)	Desirable weight (pounds)	Height (inches)	Desirable weight (pounds)
42	42.0	54	75.0
43	43.0	55	79.5
44	44.0	56	84.0
45	45.0	57	88.5
46	46.0	58	93.0
47	47.0	59	97.5
48	48.0	60	102.0
49	52.5	61	106.5
50	57.0	62	111.0
51	61.5	63	115.5
52	66.0	64	120.0
53	70.5		

According to the table, how much should you weigh?

Do you really need to lose weight? That depends on a lot of things. If you are taller or more muscular than average for your age, then you may naturally be heavier than most of your friends. If you are small-boned and petite, you will of course weigh less than others your age.

Your exact weight isn't especially important. What *is* important is what you eat and how active you are. If you eat moderate amounts of nutritious foods and get enough exercise, your weight will probably be in the right range.

Another way to tell if you are within a healthy range of weight is to find your BMI, or body mass index. The BMI includes both your height and weight. If your BMI is higher than the acceptable range, then you weigh more than someone of your height should weigh. If it is lower, than you weigh too little for your height.

BMI may sound complicated, but the math is easy. First, have someone else measure your height and weight. Then follow these steps:

1. Multiply your weight in pounds by 703.

2. Multiply your height in inches by itself. (Don't forget that a foot equals 12 inches.)

3. Divide the result of step 1 by the result of step 2. That gives you your BMI.

If even that sounds like too much work, you can use a BMI calculator on the Web. One is at www.cdc.gov/nccdphp/dnpa/bmi/calc-bmi.htm.

Now, what does your BMI mean? Use the table below to interpret your BMI.

Meaning	BMI
Underweight	Less than 18.5
Normal	18.5–24.9
Overweight	25.0–29.9
Class I obesity	30.0–34.9
Class II obesity	35.0–39.9

What is your BMI?

Is it within the normal range?

Get motivated!

You probably want to look your best, but there are many other reasons for wanting to reach an ideal weight. For instance, you may want to be able to run faster.

Think about the advantages or disadvantages of controlling your weight, and list them below.

Advantages

I will have more energy.

Disadvantages

I can't eat everything I want.

Look at your family

You probably have seen families that are all very overweight. If you have seen them at an all-you-can-eat buffet, you can guess one likely reason for their obesity! Some families simply eat too much, in restaurants and at home. They may not know enough about weight control, or they may think it's not important.

Other families have genes that incline them to gain weight. No matter how much they diet and exercise, they find it very hard to control their weight.

Look at your parents and siblings. Are they too thin, too fat, or about right?

If most of your family is overweight, it may be because everyone eats too much, or because a tendency to gain weight runs in the family. Either way, you need to be especially careful. You may have to eat less than your friends do, or exercise more. Are you thinking, "That's not fair!"? No, it's not. But life is often unfair, and you just need to deal with the cards you've been dealt.

Think about the people in your family, both those who are related to you by birth and those who live with you but are not related by birth. Circle any of the following who are overweight:

Father	Mother
Brother(s)	Sister(s)
Grandfather(s)	Grandmother(s)
Aunt(s)	Stepbrother(s)
Uncle(s)	Stepsister(s)
Stepfather	
Stepmother	

Do you see a tendency to overweight in your family?

Do you think it is inherited?

(If only those family members who are related by birth are overweight, it is likely to be inherited.)

Your family's behaviors may lead to unhealthy weights for you all. Maybe everyone is too busy and stressed to think about meals. Maybe you all eat in fast-food restaurants too often.

Can you think of a way to change those behaviors? If so, what can you do?

Do you have special problems?

In general, people can control their weight by eating carefully and exercising. That's harder for some people, though. If you have a disorder such as Type I diabetes, you have to make an extra effort to eat right.

Do you have any disorder that makes it harder for you to control your weight than it is for other people? If so, your doctor may have given you special instructions about weight control. What do you need to do?

How Can You Take Charge?

Where are you now?

Take a very honest look at yourself before starting to take charge of your weight. The best way to begin is by having someone else (such as a doctor or nurse) weigh you on a good scale. (Take your shoes off first!)

What is your present weight?

Don't be in a hurry to weigh yourself again. It's more important to form new eating and exercise habits. After you do that, your weight is likely to reach a good level. If you do lose weight, you should lose it gradually (about a pound or two per week). People who lose weight too quickly tend to gain it back.

Do you know anyone who has tried a really weird diet? They may lose a lot of weight, but it's usually only temporary. When I was your age I tried to lose weight by eating only cottage cheese at every meal. I lost a couple of pounds but gave up after a few days—and I still can't face cottage cheese! I would have been better off eating a variety of foods that included cottage cheese.

Keep track of your weight on the graph below, using a different color for your own line. The line shows the number of pounds Tom lost at the beginning of each week. At the beginning of week 6, how many pounds had he lost?

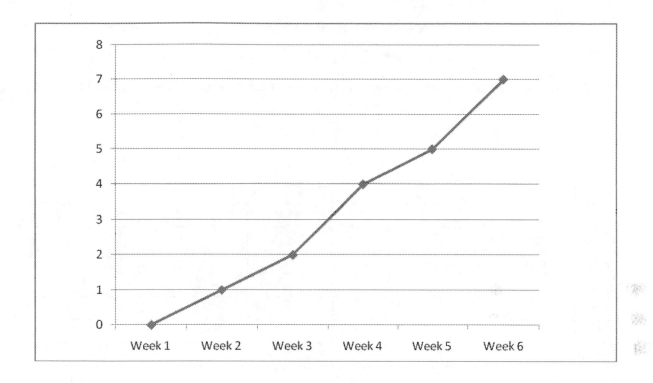

How big is a serving?

It's important to know how much a "serving" of a food is. Lists of calories in foods usually give the calories per serving. One person might think a medium-sized pizza is a serving, while another might think a one-inch slice is a serving!

How much is a "serving" of meat? Of lettuce? Of cookies? Even if you try to count your calories, it's hard to keep track if you don't know how much a serving of a food is. At the end of the book (Appendix A) is a list of common foods, showing how much of each is considered one serving. Refer to the list for this activity.

Do any of the serving sizes in Appendix A surprise you?

If you eat all the good foods you need, you may not get hungry for junk foods. For the next week, keep track of the servings of good foods you eat each day. (For the purpose of this activity, any food in Appendix A is a "good food," even if it is high in calories.) You do not need to list each food, just the group. For instance, if you eat one serving each of peanut butter, fish, and beef on Monday, you would count that as three servings in the meat group.

Food group	Servings per day						
	S	M	T	W	Th	F	S
Meat and other protein							
Fats and oils, sweets							
Vegetables							
Fruits							
Dairy foods							
Breads							

Now, compare your results with these recommendations from the U.S. Department of Agriculture (USDA) and the University of California at Los Angeles (UCLA):

Food group	Servings per day
Meat and other protein	2 to 3
Fats and oils, sweets	Eat only a little! You are getting fats from many sources, such as meat and whole milk. Many processed foods contain sugar.
Vegetables	4
Fruits	2 or 3
Dairy foods	3
Breads	3

Are you getting too little of some good foods? How can you eat more of them?

For more information about recommended foods and exercise, go to the Web site www. mypyramid.gov. This excellent site contains games and posters, also.

Ask for help!

The people around us can have a big effect on us. Maybe someone in your life bakes cookies too often. That can hurt you. Or someone is good about praising you when you do something well. That can help you.

Think about the people in your life who can help or hurt your chances of controlling your weight. Write their names in the left column in this table. Write what they do in the right column.

Name	How this person helps or hurts my chances
Mrs. Smith	Always criticizes me

Talk to at least one of the people. Ask them for more help, or ask them to stop doing something that hurts you.

How many calories are in that?

The more you know about foods, the better. Knowing something is fattening won't always stop you from eating too much of it, but often it can help you make better choices.

Go to a large supermarket and look at several cereals that you sometimes eat. Each cereal box or bin should have a Nutrition Facts label showing the number of calories and nutrients per serving. (Usually a serving of cereal is ½ cup, so if a serving is larger or smaller than that, you may need to do some calculating for this activity.) The nutrients are shown in grams, abbreviated as g. Notice what each label says, and fill in this table:

Brand and name of cereal	Calories per ½ cup	Total carbohydrates (g) per ½ cup
Post grape-nuts	*200*	*48*

Which cereal is lowest in calories?

Which cereal is lowest in total carbohydrates (carbs)?

What has this told you about these cereals? Could you choose a different cereal to help control the calories you eat?

Nutrients are the things in foods that your body needs—proteins, fats, and carbs. Proteins provide materials for building the molecules that your body needs. Fats give us stored energy. Carbs provide energy and materials for more immediate use.

All nutrients are important, but if you eat too much of any of them, the food will be stored as fat. It's especially easy to eat too many carbs, because they are less filling than fats and proteins. Proteins are used partly for building new tissues. However, large amounts of protein also are partly stored as fat. You can't safely eat too much of anything!

In general, complex carbs such as potatoes and pasta are better for you than simple carbs (sugars) such as fructose syrup, honey, or table sugar. Complex carbs are broken down more gradually in the body. Sugars are broken down for use immediately. If carbs are not used for energy, they are stored as fat. Often, breakfast cereals that appear to be good for you contain a high amount of sugars. Even complex carbs can be fattening, because they are broken down to simple carbs (sugars) in the body.

The *calories* in foods are the amount of energy you can get from the foods for moving your muscles and other activities. A gram of fat gives you 9 calories; a gram of carbs or protein gives you 4 calories. A middle-school student needs about 2500 calories/day altogether.

You can find the number of calories in almost anything if you go online and use a search engine. One helpful site is http://www.thecaloriecounter.com/. Also, you need to have a very general idea of the number of calories in common foods. For instance, a glass of lowfat milk is about 100 calories; a slice of meat or a piece of chicken, about 200 calories; a green salad, about 50 calories, a small glass of fruit juice, about 50 calories; a piece of fruit, about 100 calories; a potato, about 100 calories; a dish of ice cream, about 150 calories. All of those values depend on whether you add other things to the foods and how big the servings are!

Even if you control the carbs and calories you get from cereal, you may be adding fattening extras. Use a Web site to find out the number of calories in these extras and fill in the table:

Food	Calories
½ cup peach slices	
½ cup banana slices	
½ cup whole milk	
½ cup low fat milk	
2 tablespoons sugar	
½ cup strawberries	

Does this give you any ideas for cutting down the calories in your breakfast? What can you do to have an enjoyable breakfast with fewer calories than you get now?

Good carbs, bad carbs

We all need carbs. They provide the energy and molecules our bodies can use for building new tissues and for activities. Some carbs, called complex or "good" carbs, are helpful in controlling weight. Other carbs, called simple or "bad" carbs, are likely to cause weight gain.

Good carbs are usually made of large molecules. These are broken down gradually in the digestive system. Foods with good carbs also contain fiber. Fiber is the material that makes plant foods crunchy. Celery, for instance, has a lot of fiber. You can eat a lot of celery without gaining weight from it, and it makes you feel full. So, fiber is very useful for controlling weight. It is also good for your health in other ways.

Bad carbs are in sugary or starchy foods. These are broken down quickly in the digestive system. The products pass into the body, where they can be used as building materials and for energy. If you eat more carbs than your body needs, they are just stored as fat.

Read the following lists and think about some things you usually eat.

"Good" carbs	"Bad" carbs
carrots	cookies
apples	crackers
celery	cake
whole wheat bread and pasta	

Instead of candy, what good carb would you enjoy eating?

Instead of cookies, what good carb would you enjoy eating?

Instead of crackers, what good carb would you enjoy eating?

Instead of potato chips, what good carb would you enjoy eating?

Measure everything

For some foods, you need to measure weight or volume to see how large a serving is. If a cereal serving is ½ cup, then you should use a measuring cup to be sure you're not eating too much by mistake. If you want to eat no more than three ounces (oz.) of meat, you should weigh it on a kitchen scale.

Concentrate on measuring foods exactly for the next week. Use the following table to keep track. Each day, measure at least one food with a measuring cup or scale.

Day	I measured this food	How big or heavy was a serving?
1	*spaghetti*	*½ cup*
2		
3		
4		
5		
6		
7		

Were you surprised by how big or heavy a serving of some foods was? Which foods?

After measuring something a few times, you may be able to estimate a serving size by just looking at it. This is very useful in restaurants, especially.

Little things mean a lot

Suppose you can choose between eating two small cookies or one larger one. Which choice do you think is more fattening?

The number of calories in a cookie depends on the volume. A cookie is sort of a flattened cylinder. As you probably know, the volume of a cylinder depends on the square of the radius, or r^2. If the radius of a cookie is 1 inch, then r^2 is 1 square inch. But if the radius is 2 inches, r^2 is 4 square inches. If their thickness is the same, that means that the larger cookie has four times the volume of the smaller cookie, and four times the calories! It would be less fattening to eat two of the smaller cookies.

What's in the fridge?

Go to your refrigerator and see what foods are just sitting there waiting for you to eat them. (To save electricity, do this quickly, without holding the door open any longer than needed.) Many of the foods will be on the following list. Circle the items on the list that you find in your own refrigerator.

Soft drinks	Ice cream	Cheese
Salad greens	Bread	Butter or margarine
Frozen or fresh vegetables	Meat	Fish
Yogurt	Milk	Cake

Make another list of anything else you find in the refrigerator:

Does this give you any ideas for controlling your eating? What can you do to have more nonfattening foods available, and fewer fattening foods?

What's in the cupboard?

Even if your fridge is filled with healthy foods, you may have fattening foods in other places around the house. Do you keep snacks near the computer or TV set? Look through the kitchen cupboards or pantry. Are there cookies, candy, crackers, or other tempting foods there? If so, what did you find?

What can you do to avoid eating them?

Sleep on it

This week, keep track of the time you go to sleep each night and the time you get up each morning.

	S	M	T	W	Th	F	S
Went to sleep							
Woke up							
Number of hours slept							

At the end of the week, figure out the average number of hours of sleep you get daily. What is your average?

You should be getting 9 to 10 hours of sleep every night at your age. According to recent studies, people who get less than enough sleep are much more likely to become overweight. There may be many reasons for that. Whatever the reason is, though, you need to get enough sleep. When you go to bed, the room should be dark, and the TV and radio should be off.

Holidays

Nearly every month, some special day tempts us to eat too much. Too many chocolate bunnies at Easter or too much kugel at a Passover seder can make you gain a little bit of weight. When that is repeated on other holidays and birthdays, month after month, it becomes a lot of weight gain.

Favorite foods are part of family traditions, and you should continue to enjoy them. If you think ahead about holidays you can enjoy them without gaining weight. You can decide to have one serving of a favorite food. You might ask for a low-calorie birthday cake. After dinner you can play ball instead of watching TV.

Use the following table to list a few favorite holidays and plan how to avoid eating too much.

Holiday	Problem foods	How can I eat less of them?
Thanksgiving	Pumpkin pie	Have one small slice

Have fun!

Even if you don't eat much, you may gain weight if you spend too much time riding in a car or bus, watching TV, or reading. You need to be active part of every day.

Most days, you should get about an hour of exercise. Exercise doesn't have to be hard work. Nearly any activity that gets you moving will help you control your weight— especially if it moves you away from the cookie jar!

Think about activities you enjoy. Walking to school with friends is fun and uses up some calories. Do you like to ride your bike, swim, or play ball? Some activities are better exercise than others, but even mild exercise is better than none. You will have more fun if you do different things on different days so you won't feel bored.

The weather sometimes makes it hard to go outdoors. You can still put on boots or a parka if it is raining or snowing, but there are times when you do need to stay indoors. Be sure to plan one exercise that you can do indoors, such as jumping rope or climbing stairs.

What are some different things you can do to get exercise?

Enjoy these activities often. For the next week, keep track of what you do every day. Keep track of the amount of time you spend, too.

Day	Activity	Time spent
	Riding my bike	*30 min.*
1		
2		
3		
4		
5		
6		
7		

The USDA recommends 60 minutes of exercise a day for tweens. Are you getting that much?

Planning menus

Many families are too busy for careful meal planning. Mom or Dad may stop at a local deli or pizzeria to pick up food on the way home from work, or everyone may eat whatever is in the fridge. That can lead to fattening meals.

Planning ahead can help. Think about four simple dinners your family can eat, and write your plan in the table below. Each meal should include

- meat, fish, eggs, or both beans and rice

- a starchy vegetable, bread, or pasta

- a hot green vegetable or a green salad

- milk, no-sugar pudding, or ice cream

- fruit

An example is shown in the first row of the table.

Dinner	Meat group	Starch	Green vegetable	Milk group	Fruit
Example	pot roast with onions and carrots	potato	mixed green salad	milk	baked apple
1					
2					
3					
4					

Now, use your menus to make a grocery list. What will you need to buy for your four menus?

Grocery list	
beef	
potatoes	
salad greens	
milk	
apples	
onions	
cinnamon	
salad dressing	

Don't be bored!

One of the reasons you may eat too much is that you're feeling bored. If you're eating the same thing every day, that gets boring.

Look through some good cookbooks at home or at the library. Find some recipes that look really good. Now, challenge yourself to change them enough so the foods will also be good for you. You can substitute a no-sugar sweetener for sugar. Applesauce can substitute for butter in some recipes. It can be fun to experiment with substitutes.

In the space below, tape a copy of the original recipe you found, or write it in black ink. Use a red pen to make the changes you decided on.

"Bugaboo" foods

Everyone has some foods they can't resist. These are sometimes called "bugaboo" foods, because they are foods to fear. Max loves ice cream; Sue craves chocolate; Shawna goes crazy when she sees cookies.

What are your own "bugaboo" foods?

You need to be extremely careful about these foods. While you can have an occasional treat, if possible you shouldn't even have them in the house. It's better to buy a small candy bar or ice cream cone once in a while than to have a box of candy or carton of ice cream at home.

Let's go for a "walk"

Get a road map of your state or county and copy the part of it that includes your home. Tape the copy on the next page. Make a red X on your home. Look for a city that is about 100 miles away from your home, and use a black pencil to draw a light line from the red X to that city. Whenever you reach a goal you have set (such as not eating desserts for a week), fill in one inch of the pencil line with red ink, to show you covered 10 miles.

How far did you "walk" on your map?

How to hit the ground running

Research shows that people who eat a good breakfast eat less later in the day. In fact, someone once said that to control weight, it's best to "breakfast like a king, lunch like an ordinary citizen, and dine like a pauper." Many of us do just the opposite. We rush to school or work without having a good breakfast. Then we feel tired and hungry by mid-morning, so we eat a sweet roll or other junk food. At lunchtime we may either eat too much or too little (if there is something else to do at that time). Around four o'clock we feel hungry again, so we may eat a candy bar or cookie. By the time we have dinner, we have had a lot of calories, but little good food. So, we tend to eat a large dinner.

For the next few days, keep track of everything you eat, including snacks, in the following table. If you have a good breakfast, write a "K" (for king) in that column. If not, write a "P" (for pauper) there. "C" stands for "citizen."

Day	Breakfast	Lunch	Dinner	Snacks
Example	*P*	*C*	*K*	*K*
1				
2				
3				
4				

What sort of eating pattern do you have? Can you think of some ways of improving it?

Hidden dangers

Sometimes people try very hard to keep from gaining weight, but they fail. In many cases that's because they are kidding themselves. They may eat in a sushi bar because the food seems nonfattening, but they eat too much of it, or they choose the wrong kinds.

Salad bars look like a good solution to weight gain, and they can be. But if you add a lot of salad dressing, bacon bits, and cheese to a tossed salad, it's not a diet meal any longer. Some salad bars have guacamole, sour cream, and other additions that are high-calorie. Even lowfat, no-sugar yogurt can get you if you add candy toppings.

Think about possible hidden dangers in the foods you eat. How can you avoid them?

Danger	How I can avoid it
mayo on my sandwiches	substitute mustard for mayo

Postpone extras

Sometimes just slowing down can help you eat less. Do you ever find that if you postpone eating something for a while, you don't crave it as much?

For a few days, try postponing some snacks and desserts. Keep track in this table:

Kind of food	How long did you wait to eat it?
candy	*1 hour*

Did this activity help you? Did you find that after postponing a snack, you no longer wanted it?

Seeing through ads

This activity will help you understand how advertising may influence what you think or do. First, look through some of the magazines you see often. Ads are powerful persuaders! An ad for a car, for example, may show a happy family gathering in the mountains. The ad promises that if you buy a certain kind of car, you will automatically be happy in some ways.

Collect at least ten ads that try to persuade the reader to buy non-food items such as clothing or cars, and use them to fill in this table:

What product is being advertised?   What does the ad promise?

Some ads for foods make false promises, too. An ad for a hamburger may show a bunch of teenagers having a good time on a beach or at a swimming pool. All of them are wearing swimsuits, and they look great. They happen to be eating hamburgers, too. If you see that ad enough times, you may be more likely to buy that kind of hamburger.

Cut out ten ads for food or drinks. Fill out this table, based on those ads:

What food or drink is being advertised?   What does the ad promise?

Were any of the ads for foods or drinks you ordinarily consume? Does understanding an ad make you more likely to resist a food that is fattening or not nutritious?

Picture yourself

Look through some magazines or clothing catalogs, and find a picture of someone you'd like to resemble. (Don't pick a too-skinny model, or one who behaves badly!) Cut the picture out and tape it in the space below or on your fridge. Looking at the picture once in a while may help you control your eating.

At the mall

A day at the mall can mean hanging out with family or friends and eating too much, as well as shopping. But it doesn't have to be that way. You can have fun without doing anything that will make you gain weight.

First, think about how much walking you do at the mall. Do you or your parents try to park near the stores where you plan to spend time? Instead, think about where you could park that would be as far away as possible. In the space below, draw a sketch of the mall where you usually go. Then use a red pencil to show a parking space near the outside of the mall. Draw a dotted red line from the parking space to various places where you may want to go.

Did this give you any ideas for increasing your walking time at the mall?

Now, think about the mall's restaurants or food court. Which one has the least fattening food? Can you persuade your family or friends to go there? If not, where will you probably eat?

Plan what you will eat. What can you have that won't be fattening?

You may even want to carry a lunch with you, and just buy some milk or diet soda to drink. Whatever you do, you can have something for lunch that isn't fattening, and you can avoid junk foods.

Trying something new

Have you ever tried eating tofu? Some people are afraid to try it, and they miss out on some delicious meals as a result. Tofu itself is a bland, white food made of soybeans. It has very little taste in itself but picks up flavors from other ingredients.

To find out if you might enjoy tofu, get a small amount of the firm kind from a health-food store or the produce section of a supermarket. Cut it into cubes about the size of sugar cubes, put them into a frypan, and soak them in your favorite barbecue sauce. *Have an adult watch* while you fry the cubes lightly on the stove. Put a tooth pick in each one, and use the picks to hold the cubes as you eat them.

Did you enjoy the tofu?

Can you think of other ways you might eat it?

If you liked tofu, watch for it in restaurants and food stores. It is used often in spicy Asian foods, for instance. Because it is low in fat and sugar and has few calories, it is very good diet food.

Here is my own recipe for using tofu. You or an adult may enjoy trying it. It tastes a little like banana bread.

Applesauce Bread or Muffins (large loaf or 12 muffins)

Set oven at 350 ºF for bread or 400 ºF for muffins. Lightly oil a loaf pan or muffin tin.

Mix:

½ cup mashed tofu

1 cup unsweetened applesauce

3 eggs

2 cups Bisquick

¾ cup Splenda sweetener

1/3 cup vegetable oil

½ teaspoon vanilla

1/3 cup wheat germ or crushed walnuts

Pour into the pan. Bake 60 minutes.

Planning fast foods

Go to your favorite fast-food restaurant. Before ordering anything, look carefully at the menu and answer these questions:

- What do you usually eat here?

- Is there a smaller version of what you usually eat on the menu?

- Is there a salad on the menu that looks good?

- Can you order the salad without any dressing?

- Can you split an order of something with a friend?

- What other ways can you think of to eat less in your favorite restaurant?

Many people eat while they are watching TV, reading, or using a computer. It's easy to eat too much without even realizing what you're doing.

Think about some of those times when you eat too much and then fill in the chart.

I eat too much while I _____. I can _____ instead of eating.

watch TV *draw or paint*

Did you think of some good substitutes for eating? Maybe you can get up and walk around for a few minutes every half hour or so. Maybe you can eat some good snacks, such as carrot sticks or an apple, instead of buttered popcorn or candy. Whatever you do should be easy for you. You should enjoy your snacks.

Working off calories

Exercise is as important as dieting for weight control. Here are some values for the amount of energy used by some activities:

Low:

Dancing	150 calories/hour
Cycling	250 calories/hour
Playing baseball	250 calories/hour

Moderate:

Brisk walking	350 calories/hour
Stair climbing	300 calories/hour

Strenuous:

Swimming laps	550 calories/hour

Very strenuous:

Running (1 block per minute)	750 calories/hour
Skiing	750 calories/hour

(Note: These are very rough values. The number of calories you use depends on your weight and how vigorously you exercise.)

Choose some activity you enjoy. Each day for a week, try to use up at least 100 calories by exercising. Keep track in the following table:

Date	Kind of activity	Calories used

Total for week

How many calories did you use this week by exercising?

Can you think of some other activity that might be useful for burning up calories? What is it?

The price of fast food

Sometimes people eat fast food because it doesn't cost much. Make a list of the things that are needed to make a typical fast-food meal—for example, a cheeseburger, fries, and soft drink. Be sure to include buns, lettuce, and other ingredients. Now take the list to a grocery store and find out how much the items cost. (Probably you will have to "buy" enough for six or eight people.) Fill in the following table with the list and prices:

Item	Cost per package
ground beef	*$3*

Now use the table to figure out the cost of the meal for each person. For ground beef the cost is $3/pound, so that works out to $0.50 per serving.

How much would it cost you to buy one meal at a fast food restaurant?

How much would it cost to make the meal at home?

Even if you can save money by cooking them yourself, restaurant-made fast foods are often convenient. However, homemade meals have other advantages. What are they?

You know exactly what is in them.

Your own trail mix

Do you ever eat trail mix? Many people carry trail mix with them when they are hiking, or they eat it as a snack at other times. Trail mix contains nuts, seeds, and other nutritious ingredients. But trail mix can be high in calories, even if it is good for you. It may also contain candy or other sugary ingredients. These can be high in calories without adding much nutrition.

Examine the table below, which shows the calories per gram (g) of some typical trail mix ingredients. (A gram is about the weight of one peanut.)

Ingredient	Calories/g
Peanuts	6
Raisins	4
Candy	5
Walnuts	7
Almonds	6
Sunflower seeds	6
Wheat cereal	4

Circle the ingredients you really like. Draw a line through any you don't like. Now, think about how to make your own trail mix—one you will enjoy, but it won't be as fattening as some others are.

What will you put into your trail mix?

How did you make it as nutritious and nonfattening as possible?

Walking

Now that you have some good trail mix, you can hit the trail! Start with an easy walk of about a mile (eight city blocks). You can plan the hike with a map. Copy a local map, or draw it yourself. Then use a colored pencil to draw a circle on it that begins and ends at the same place. Use the map's key to figure out how long the line should be, so that when you reach the starting point again you have covered a mile. Take the map with you. If you are walking alone, be sure to tell an adult where you are going and how long you will be gone.

Always carry a small bottle of water with you when you hike. In hot weather, especially, you will get thirsty. You can keep it in a large pocket or a backpack. If you plan to walk very far, take a small package of trail mix, too.

Try to walk at a rate of about 3 miles per hour. Walking a mile at that rate should take you about 20 minutes.

You can work up to longer walks gradually. Don't try to walk much faster or farther. The important thing is to walk often, preferably every day. Daily walking can be a lifelong, enjoyable activity. Some people like to wear a pedometer to help them keep track of how far they walk each day. A pedometer isn't really necessary, but you may enjoy using one.

To get started, fill in this table:

Date   Miles walked

Walking your dog

Do you have a dog? Dogs need to be walked every day, and they are good companions. Some dogs walk fast enough for you to get exercise while you walk them. Other dogs stroll along slowly, sniffing every blade of grass.

Whichever kind of dog you have, walking it every day is good for you. Even if you don't get a lot of exercise, you are moving.

If you don't have a dog of your own, you may want to offer to walk someone else's dog. They will appreciate the help, you will have the pleasure of walking the dog, and you won't have to feed it or take it to the vet!

In the following space, write a paragraph about the dog you walk. Describe the kind of dog, how often you walk it, and whether walking it gives you exercise. Draw a picture of the dog, or tape a photo into the book.

Don't get hungry!

When you're really hungry, you're more likely to eat anything in sight. If you eat a small snack between meals, you won't be likely to eat too much at mealtime. The danger in snacking is that you may be tempted to eat junk food, such as cookies or potato chips. These are very high in calories and don't satisfy your hunger for very long. Some snacks are good for satisfying your hunger, though. Some people like to snack on apples or no-sugar pudding, for instance. Water can be a good snack, too. Sometimes when we feel hungry, we're actually thirsty.

Think about some low-calorie snacks. They should be foods or drinks you enjoy. If you are taking them with you someplace, they should be easy to carry. What are some low-calorie snacks you can take anywhere?

What can you say?

Sometimes your family and friends can make it harder for you to control your weight. They may not understand what you need to do. If you don't want to be rude, you may find yourself accepting second helpings of food, or doing something else that is bad for you.

It helps to plan ahead and think about what you can say to people. For instance, if you're walking to school and a friend's mom offers you a ride, you might smile and say, "No, thanks! I need to walk a mile today."

Think about what you might say in the following situations, and write your answers in the table.

If this happens	You can do or say this:
Someone offers you a dessert, but you don't want it.	
A friend says that eating something just once can't hurt you.	
A friend wants to watch TV or play a video game, and you need to get some exercise.	

Try to think of some other problems friends and family members might cause. Does it help you to practice what you can do or say?

How Are You Doing?

After a few weeks of doing the activities in this book, you should be taking charge of your eating and exercising. You may have started to lose some weight, too. Weigh yourself, or have someone else weigh you, as you did earlier. What do you weigh now?

Do you have more energy than you did a few weeks ago?

Try again

Answer the following questions—you'll recognize them from the beginning of the book.

1.   What is your favorite snack?

2.   If a 2" cookie has 100 calories, how many calories are in a 4" cookie of the same kind and thickness?

3.   How far can you walk in 20 minutes if you walk 3 miles per hour?

4.   How much sleep do people your age need every night?

5.   What is the least fattening cereal you know about?

6.   Why is tofu a healthy food?

7.   How much milk should you drink every day?

8.   Does swimming or walking use up more calories a minute?

9.   Do you eat breakfast every day?

Are your answers the same now?

Reward yourself

Feeling and looking healthier is a good reward for eating well and exercising, but you can give yourself other rewards that will help you take charge of your weight. Aleesha's mom wanted to help her walk more often, so every time Aleesha finished walking 10 miles, she got a small reward. One time it was a special magazine. Another time it was a tube of lip gloss. Looking forward to the rewards helped Aleesha walk more, but her greatest reward was losing a few pounds.

Fill in this table with the things you plan to do and the rewards you can give yourself.

What I plan to do	How I'll reward myself
lose 5 pounds	*buy a special tee shirt*

Look better, feel better

No one should be too concerned about their looks. What a person is like inside is much more important. However, we need to pay some attention to how we look. Other people may judge us by our appearance. Also, when we look good, we tend to feel good about ourselves. When we feel good, we find it easier to take good care of our health and appearance. It's a continual cycle of look good → feel good → look good.

The opposite is true, too. When we look bad, we can start to feel sad or grumpy. That makes it hard to take care of ourselves. It's a continual cycle of look bad → feel bad → look bad.

How we dress affects how we look. For this activity, look through some online sites, magazine ads, or clothing catalogs. Choose something you'd like to wear, such as a swimsuit or exercise outfit. Print or cut out the picture and tape it in the space below. You may want to buy the clothing now, or use it as a reward after carrying out some of the other activities in the book.

A Final Word

I hope carrying out the exercises in this book has helped you to control your weight. It's not easy, and you may need to work at it all your life. I was a fat child and teenager many years ago. Being fat made me unhappy and was bad for my health. As an adult, I learned how to control my weight while eating the foods I needed to be healthy. Losing weight has made my adult life much happier than it would have been if I had stayed fat, and I want you to gain from what I learned. The earlier in life you take charge of your weight, the better.

Carol Leth Stone

P.O. Box 9

Pollock Pines, CA 95726

StoneCottage2@juno.com

For Further Reading

These books are written for parents and teachers. Tweens may want to look at them for recipes and more information.

Bean, Anita. *Awesome Foods for Active Kids.* Alameda, CA: Hunter House Inc., 2006.

Kelly, Evelyn. *Obesity.* Westport, CT: Greenwood Press, 2006.

Neufeld, Naomi. *Kid Shape: A Practical Prescription for Raising Healthy, Fit Children.* Nashville, TN: Rutledge Hill Press, 2004.

Pollan, Michael. *The Omnivore's Dilemma.* NY: Penguin Press, 2006.

Stone, Carol. *Cooking without Sugar.* Lincoln, NB: iUniverse, Inc., 2002.

_____. *The Basics of Biology.* Westport, CT: Greenwood Press, 2004.

Appendix A: Calories in Some Foods

The calories in these foods refer to the foods themselves, without any additions. For instance, the mashed potatoes do not contain any butter or sour cream!

Food group	Food	Size of a serving	Calories in a serving
Bread	Bread	1 slice	80
	Diet bread	2 slices	80
	Corn or flour tortilla	1 (6″ diameter)	80
	Most cold cereals	1 ounce (¼–1 cup)	80
	Cooked cereal	½ cup	80
	Cooked rice	½ cup	80
	Cooked pasta	½ cup	80
	Popped light popcorn	3 cups	80
Vegetables	Corn	½ cup cooked corn or 1 medium ear	80
	Cooked mixed vegetables	½ cup	80
	Baked potato	3 ounces (1 small)	80
	Cooked mashed potatoes	½ cup	80
	Cooked squash	1 cup	80
	Cooked yam or sweet potato	½ cup	80
	Cooked or canned beans (plain)	½ cup	80
	Raw leafy vegetables	1 cup	25
	Raw nonleafy vegetables	1 cup	25
Fruit	Apple	1 small (4 ounces)	60
	Banana	1 small (4″)	60
	Blueberries	¾ cup	60
	Whole strawberries	1¼ cup	60
	Raspberries	1 cup	60

	Cantaloupe	1 cup	60
	Watermelon	¼ cup	60
	Peach	1 medium	60
	Grapefruit	½ medium	60
	Grapes or cherries	12	60
	Raisins	2 Tbsp	60
	Orange	1 medium	60
	100% fruit juice	4–6 ounces	60
Dairy	Nonfat or 1% milk	8 ounces (1 cup)	90
	1% plain yogurt	8 ounces (1 cup)	90
	Grated parmesan	3 ounces	100
	Lowfat cheese	3 ounces	100
	Nonfat frozen yogurt	½ cup	80
Meat	White meat of chicken	3 ounces	100
	Dark meat of chicken	3 ounces	225
	Light tofu	¼ cup	100
	Fish	3 ounces	100
	Shellfish	3 ounces	100
	Nonfat cheese or cottage cheese	3 ounces	100
	Canned tuna in oil	3 ounces	100
	Fried chicken or fish	3 ounces	225
	Lean beef	3 ounces	165
	Pork	3 ounces	225
	Ground beef (hamburger)	3 ounces	225
	Egg	1 large	80
	Mozzarella or feta cheese	3 ounces	225
	Most cheeses	1 ounce	225
	Regular tofu	3 ounces	225
	Hot dog	3 ounces	300
	Bacon	3 slices	100
Fats and oils	Olive, canola, peanut oils	1 tsp	45
	Olives, stuffed	8 large	45

	Most nuts	½ oz	45
	Pecan or walnut halves	4	45
	Margarine	1 tsp	45
	Mayonnaise	1 tsp	45
	Salad dressing	1 tbsp	45

About the Author

Carol Leth Stone is a science writer and editor who has authored or contributed to numerous programs for science and health education. She has done graduate work in biology and earned a Ph.D. from the Stanford University School of Education. Because she was overweight as a child and teenager, she has a special interest in helping young people learn to control their weight before it becomes a problem for them. Today she lives in the forested Sierra Nevada mountains in northern California. When she is not traveling in her RV, she uses it as a writing studio.